ERKINBEK DZHAMANBAEV, D.M.

PANCHAKARMA – A PRACTICAL GUIDE
By Dr.Erkin

Part 1. Preparatory/Preliminary Procedures
(Poorvakarma)

- If we don't have the power to choose where we come from,
we can still choose where we go from there.
"The Perks of Being a Wallflower". Stephen Chbosky

INTRODUCTION

Ayurveda deals with the preventive and curative aspects of health. It comes under the classification of Traditional Medicine (TM) as per the specifications of W.H.O and is in the process of acquiring international recognition.

Ayurveda emphasizes complete eradication of the disease and for that Shodhana (Ayurvedic bio purification) therapy is used. Shodhana therapy eradicates the vitiated Dosha from the root and minimizes the chances of recurrence of the disease. Panchakarma is the five Shodhana (bio purification) procedures having a different scope of action. The Panchakarma procedures when carried out as per classical guidelines with all reparatory procedures and post-care removes all toxins and morbid Dosha from the body, revitalizes the body, prevent aging and degenerative changes and promotes longevity of life. Panchakarma is a very famous and esteemed procedure of Ayurveda. The pharmacodynamics of many processes are not been explained yet in modern terminology but Ayurveda has an explanation for every activity of Panchakarma in its terminology.

Panchakarma a specialty of Kaya Chikitsa (Internal Medicine) Ayurveda section presents a unique approach of Ayurveda with specially designed five procedures of internal purification of the body through the nearest possible route. Such purification allows the biological system to return to homeostasis and to rejuvenate rapidly and also facilitates the desired pharmacokinetic effect of medicines administered thereafter. Panchakarma provides a comprehensive therapy role as a promotive, preventive, curative & rehabilitative procedure.

Panchakarma is not merely bio-purificatory therapy as it is understood, but also has a wider range of therapeutics such as replenishing, depleting, rejuvenating therapies, etc.

Ayurveda emphasizes preventative and healing therapies along with various methods of purification and rejuvenation. Ayurveda is more than a mere healing system. It is a science and art of appropriate living which helps to achieve longevity. It can also guide every individual in the prevention of disease and long term maintenance of health.

To achieve this balanced state of body, mind, and consciousness, Ayurveda prescribes Panchakarma Therapy for the cleansing of body toxins, deranged Dosha and Mala.

Besides their application in the treatment of the disease, they are also used as preparatory measures before the institution of surgery and also before administration of rejuvenation therapy, virility therapy, and palliative medicines. But Panchakarma, the purification therapy expounded in Ayurveda is perhaps the most misunderstood of all the Ayurveda practices. Due to ignorance, it is often perceived as just another system of oil massage.

Definition

As the name suggests, "Pancha" in Sanskrit stands for Five and Karma are the therapeutic measures, therefore Panchakarma means five types of therapeutic measures. These are performed for the purification of the body and Ayurveda considers it necessary before the start of any other therapy. As a cloth needs to be clean and washed before dyeing it with a new color, otherwise the cloth will not be dyed properly. Similarly, the body needs to be purified before any treatment so that it grasps the new colors of youthfulness, health, and vigor. Most of the time, Panchakarma is an end in itself rather than a prelude to other therapeutic measures because the cleansing alone is sufficient for the eradication of many disorders.

The Panchakarma therapy of Ayurveda is comprised of five types of advanced treatment for the evacuation of vitiated Dosha from the body. These practices are extremely helpful in relieving deep seated diseases as well as maintaining and improving physical and mental health.

Sodhana and Shamana Chikitsa - two essential treatment types for Ayurveda

Ayurveda treatment is branched into two wings – Sodhana (Purification treatment) and Shamana (Alleviating treatment).

Sodhana Chikitsa

Treatments begin with Sodhana Chikitsa. This is to discard the internal cause factors of the disease. The continuous metabolic process causes the quantified formation of toxic bioproducts in the body. The toxins cause vitiation of Doshas and Dhatus resulting in the impairment of systems.

In Sodhana Chikitsa five therapeutic methods (Panchakarma) are employed as under:

1. Vamana (emesis therapy). Oral medicines are given to induce vomiting.
2. Virechana (purgation therapy). Oral medicines are given to induce purgation.
3. Nasyam (nasal medication). Medicated oil or powder is administered through the nostrils.
4. Vasty (enema therapy). Medicated oil or decoction is administered through the anus.
5. Rakthamoksham (bloodletting therapy). Impure blood is drained out through various means.

Shamana Chikitsa

Shamana Chikitsa - is the alleviating therapy that is done after Sodhana Chikitsa. Herbal medicines are administered orally and externally to correct the functions of Doshas, Dhatus, Malas, and Agni and discard the ailments and immunize the body.

According to Ayurveda, when the vitiated Dosha interacts with Dhatu, the disease process is initiated. If this interaction is mild then it can be managed by pacifying (Shamana) measures of treatment. But if the interaction is severe or chronic then those accumulated Dosha in the form of wastes or toxins have to be eliminated and for this purpose, five measures of bio-purification (Shodhana) are used.

Panchakarma therapy is considered better than any other therapy because it eliminates the vitiated Dosha out of the body, so there is a little chance of recurrence of the disease. On the other hand, the Dosha pacified by Shamana treatment may recur by a little reason. Thus Panchakarma is mainly a treatment of major and chronic diseases caused by excessive vitiation of Dosha.

Besides, Panchakarma therapy is also useful for the prevention of diseases. E.g. if Vamana therapy is taken just before the beginning of the spring, the incidence of Kapha disorders are prevented to a large extent. Similarly, purgation therapy received in autumn and Basti in the rainy season prevents Pitta and Vata disorders respectively. Observing the respective seasonal regimen also prevents the diseases caused by vitiation of Dosha as well as retards the aging process.

Rasayana and Vajikarana are two therapies for the promotion of health. But before the administration of both of these therapies, it is mandatory to purify the body by Panchakarma to get the optimal benefits of these health-promoting measures. In this way, Panchakarma is important for both prevention as well as treatment of the diseases.

Panchakarma has always performed in three stages preparatory/pre-operative procedure, main/operative procedure, and post-operative procedure. The patient who opts for any one of the five therapies has to invariably undergo all the three stages or steps.

Three steps of Panchakarma

1. **Poorva Karma (preparation for purification):** Deepana, Pachana (neutralize Ama), Snehana, Swedana
2. **Pradhana Karma (main procedures):** Vamana, Virechana, Basti, Nasya, Raktamokshana, Anuvasana, Asthapana,
3. **Pashchat Karma (post cleansing procedures):** Samsarjana Krama (dieting), Rasayana, Pathya Patana Shamana

Preparatory/Preliminary Procedures (Poorvakarma)

Before the administration of actual bio-purificatory therapy, there is a need to prepare the body in prescribed methods to encourage the body to let go of the toxins.

<u>**Preparatory procedures include:**</u>
- Deepana (Kindling of digestive fire)
- Pachana (Digestion)
- Snehana (Oleation)
- Swedana (Sudation)

Deepana & Pachana do kindling of fire and digestion of metabolic toxins respectively. Ghee or oil is given daily for three to seven days. Snehana loosens the toxins & helps in the separation of toxins from tissues. It also makes the superficial and deep tissues soft and supple. Swedana is sudation or sweating and is given for 1 to 3 days after the massage. Swedana liquefies the toxins and helps in the movement of toxins into the gastrointestinal tract. After three to seven days of Snehana, massage, and sudation the Dosha (bio-humors) is liquefied and brought to GIT. Then specific Panchakarma therapy is administered according to the involvement of bio-humor.

Snehana Karma: Medicated oil and medicated ghee are administered internally and externally in various methods such as Sneha Panam, Abhyanga Massage, Sirodhara, Shirobasti, Pizhichil, etc.

Swedana Karma: The methods adopted are Njavarakizhi, Elakizhi, Choorna Sweda, Steam bath, hot herbal bath, etc.

As we know, Dosha and Mala actively participate in physiological functions. Whenever due to some etiology, the Dosha deranges from their normal function they become hazardous to the body and it becomes necessary to either correct them or eliminate them. Panchakarma measures are adopted to eliminate them from the body but it is not as simple as it sounds. As the Dosha is operational at the macro as well as a micro-level of the body functions, they are present in each cell of the body and resultant pathology is also impregnated at the cellular level. It is not possible to eliminate the Dosha without proper loosening and separating them from the cells and tissues. Purification measures adopted without proper loosening, agglomerating and channelizing of the Dosha may be a failure and can also harm the healthy tissue. Before the performance of bio-purification, it is necessary to make a patient biologically ready to expel the accumulated morbid material and this process is known as Purvakarma.

The purpose of Purvakarma is to loosen the morbid Dosha and toxins to agglomerate the fragmented Dosha for the ease of removal to channelize them into gastro-intestinal tract or nasopharynx (as per the site of disease) to facilitate their removal from natural routs and to strengthen the body to withstand the stress of Panchakarma therapy.

Pashchata karma: Post Purification measures of Panchakarma

After bio-purification, digestive fire/Bio-fire (Agni) & strength of the body becomes weak. So to restore the strength of digestive fire & body special dietetic regimen is advised. Also, some restrictions related to food & behavior are advised to the person who undergone Panchakarma.

Includes dietetic regimen, rejuvenation, and administration of palliative medicine.
After performing the major Karma particularly emesis and purgation, due to the exertion the digestive Agni becomes weak. To avoid Agni related complications and to enkindle the Agni to its full capacity, a regime about diet and behavior called "Samsarjana Krama" is followed for a stipulated

period. Pashchata Karma restores the normal strength of the body, restores Agni and also makes sure that the Dosha does not relapse.

Timing effect
There is a false assumption in the society about Ayurvedic treatment that it takes a long time to show results. But Panchakarma is a rapidly acting therapy that can be used in emergency conditions to eliminate the severely aggravated Dosha. In the main process of Vamana Karma, emesis starts within 48 minutes of administration of a drug and Niruha Basti (herbal decoction) also comes out within 48 minutes of administration. Similarly, the process of Virechana is completed within a few hours and the whole process of Nasya is completed within one hour.

Pradhana Karma (main course): Panchakarma (Five Major Bio-Purification Therapies)

1. Vamana (Therapeutic vomiting or emesis)
2. Virechana (Purgation)
3. Asthapana and Anuvasana Basti (Therapeutic Enema, decoction & oil)
4. Nasya (Elimination of toxins through the nose/errhine therapy)
5. Raktamokshana (Bloodletting)

Vamana (Emesis Therapy)

When there is congestion in the lungs causing repeated attacks of bronchitis, colds, cough or asthma, the Ayurvedic treatment is therapeutic vomiting, to eliminate the Kapha. Therapeutic vomiting is mainly indicated in chronic asthma, chronic sinusitis, and skin diseases involving the upper part of the body, diabetes, chronic cold, lymphatic congestion, chronic indigestion, and edema.

Virechana (Purgation Therapy)

When excess Pitta is accumulated in the gall bladder, liver, and small intestine, it tends to result in rashes, skin inflammation, acne, chronic recurrent fever, biliary vomiting, nausea, and jaundice. Ayurvedic literature suggests in these conditions the administration of therapeutic purgation.

Basti (Therapeutic Enema)

Vata is the main factor involved in pathogenesis (disease). If one can control Vata through the use of Basti, then it is easier to treat the root cause of the vast majority of diseases. Vata is the motive force behind the elimination and retention of feces, urine, bile, and other excreta. Vata is mainly located in the large intestine, but bone tissue (Asthi Dhatu) is also a site for Vata. Hence the medication administered rectally affects Asthi Dhatu. The mucus membrane of the colon is related to the bone tissue.

Therefore, any medication given rectally goes into the deeper tissues, like bones, and pacifies Vata disorders. Ayurvedic Basti involves the introduction of herbal concoctions of sesame oil and certain herbal preparations in a liquid medium into the rectum. Basti is the most effective treatment in Vata disorders. It relieves constipation, distention, chronic fever, cold, sexual disorders, kidney stones, heart pain, backache, sciatica and other pains in the joints. Many other Vata disorders such as arthritis, rheumatism, gout, muscle spasms, and headaches may also be treated with Basti.

Nasya (Errhine Therapy)
The nose is the gateway to the brain. The nasal administration of medication is called Nasya. An excess of bio-humors accumulated in the sinus, throat, nose, or head areas is eliminated through the nose.

Prana, life force as nerve energy, enters the body through the breath taken in through the nose. Prana is in the brain and maintains sensory and motor functions. Prana also governs mental activities, memory, concentration, and intellectual activities. Deranged Prana creates defective functioning of all these activities and produces headaches, convulsions, loss of memory and reduced sensory perception. Thus nasal administration, Nasya is indicated for nervous system disorders, sinus congestion, migraine headaches, convulsions, and certain eye and ear problems.

Raktamokshana (Bloodletting therapy)
Toxins present in the gastrointestinal tract are absorbed into the blood and circulated throughout the body. The metabolic waste products are not eliminated properly & the free radicals produced by them are the basic cause of repeated infections, hypertension, and certain other circulatory conditions. This includes repeated attacks of skin disorders such as urticaria, rashes, herpes, eczema, acne, leukoderma, chronic itching or hives. In these conditions, along with internal medication, elimination of the toxins and purification of the blood is necessary. Raktamokshana is also indicated for cases of enlarged liver, spleen, and gout. Removing a small amount of blood from the vein purifies the Pitta bio-humor. Bloodletting also stimulates the spleen & liver which in turn stimulates the immune system. Toxins are neutralized enabling radical cures in many blood born disorders.

CLASSIFICATION OF PANCHAKARMA

Preventive, Promotive and Curative

Preventive and Promotive Panchakarma subdivided into 6 types viz. Regular, Complete, Purificatory, Rejuvenation, Relaxation & Immune booster.

a) Regular: therapies such as oil massage, medicated smoking, oil pulling, etc. used daily
b) Complete: administration of Vamana etc.5 therapies
c) Purificatory: administration of Vamana & Virechana
d) Rejuvenation: administration of Vamana, virechana and then Rasayana Basti course for 30 days
e) Relaxation: Massage, Shirodhara, etc.
f) Immune enhancing: Administration of Vamana, Virechana and then Rasayana Basti course for 30 days

g) Curative Panchakarma: Disease-specific Panchakarma

Classical & traditional (Keraliyan)

Keraliyan Panchakarma therapies are the modified & sophisticated external Snehana & Swedana therapies told in the classics. These therapies gained global recognition due to their high therapeutic efficacy in healthy & diseased and also their use in resorts, spas, and restaurants. All the Keraliyan Panchakarma therapies will be described in detail later.

Mode of action
1. Somatic level: Metabolism, Immunity, Free radical elimination
2. Psychic level: Antistress, relaxation of mind
3. Neuro-endocrine level: normalization of secretory activities

Panchakarma does not just eliminate disease-causing toxins but also revitalizes the tissues. Hence it is called rejuvenation therapy. In today's world more and more people are falling victim to the adverse effects of stress and anxiety, which is leading to diseases like improper digestion, lack of sleep, allergies, heart diseases, diabetes, chronic fatigue, cancer, osteoporosis, etc.

These diseases are caused mainly due to deeply seated toxins. Panchakarma eliminates these toxins from the body, allowing permanent healing of tissues, channels, digestion, and mental functions. Panchakarma is not only good for alleviating disease but is also a useful therapy in maintaining excellent health. Ayurveda advises undergoing Panchakarma during seasonal changes to purify the body, improve digestion and to improve the metabolic processes.

If the Dosha (bio-humors) are vitiated beyond a particular level, they give rise to various endotoxins, which tend to be accumulated in the minute channels. These are beyond the level of pacification and hence need to be eliminated or removed from the body. In such cases, bio-purificatory therapy is indicated.

FUNDAMENTAL PRINCIPLES OF PANCHAKARMA

Basic principles

A. Excitation of bio-humors (Dosha), by Snehana (oleation) and Swedana (sudation).

B. Expulsion of bio-humors, mainly by Vamana, but all 5 therapies can be needed

C. Pacification of Dosha, achieved by Snehana, Swedana, Basti & Nasya.

D. Nourishment of tissues & increasing the immunity, achieved by Snehana, Basti, Nasya

E. Depleting the tissues, by Swedana, Vamana, and all 5 therapies

F. Post-Panchakarma dietetic regimen (Sansarjana Kramas), this is Peyadi Krama, Tarpanadi Krama, and Rasa Sansarjana⬚

G. Behavioral and dietetic restriction

Importance of Panchakarma

1. The Ayurvedic classics categorically emphasized that bio-purificatifiion (Shodhana) of both body and mind is essential pre-requisite for the administration of Rasayana therapy because if channels (Srotas) are not clean, the rejuvenation effect will not be achieved in the same way as the unclean cloth does not stain properly with color. Bio-purification is essential to obtain the effects of rejuvenation and aphrodisiac action of the drug. Without bio-purification, they are administered then they will be having less effect. For proper attainment of rejuvenation effect, cleansing of channels (Srotoshodhana) and enhancement of the biological fire (Agnideepana) is required, which are effectively done by the bio-purificatory therapy.

2. The bio-humors eliminated by bio-purificatory therapy never recur but those pacified by dieting (Langhana), digestive (Pachana), etc. may recur.

3. Benefits of bio-purification therapy as follows. Vitiated biohumors are eliminated, the power of digestion and metabolism is enhanced, diseases are cured, normal health is restored, sense organs, mind, intelligence, and complexion become clear; gain of strength, plumpness, offspring, and virility occur; a person is not affected by old age and lives long without any disease.

4. The unique feature of the Panchakarma therapy is to destroy the disease from the root level, in some way if bio-humors are not destroyed from the root, they again cause diseases. Bio-purification therapy acts on the root sites of bio-humor and removes them from the body so that there is no further nutrition to the other sites of bio-humor leading to a healthy condition. Thus Panchakarma is a radical treatment.

5. If bio-purification is administered properly it pacifies the disease, destroys the disease and increases the strength and health.

Utility of Panchakarma

- Panchakarma plays a vital role in the preservation, maintenance, & conservation of health & promotion of longevity. They form a part in the regimen of preventive medicine (Svastha Vritta) indicated as prophylactic measures in the context of epidemics and pan epidemics.
- These measures are indicated as preparatory procedures before the administration of rejuvenation therapy (Rasayana) & aphrodisiac therapy (Vajikarana).
- All diseases occur due to suppression and forceful expulsion of natural urges, Panchakarma is the best treatment for the diseases caused by the suppression of natural urges (Vega Dharana). Suppression of natural urges affects gastrointestinal motility and

continence of sphincters and later neuro-humoral control of glands.
- Weak digestive fire (Mandagni) is the cause of many diseases. For the correction of digestive fire (Agni), Panchakarma is the best treatment.
- In diseases due to overnutrition (Santarpanajanya Roga) elimination of humor (Doshavasecana) is indicated. Most of the diseases are due to weak digestive fire. So Panchakarma therapy is best for the correction of Agni. In a person with disturbed homeostasis, there is impaired anabolism and catabolism resulting in decreased nutrition and immunity impaired excretion of waste products leading to the collection of metabolic waste. All these lead to the formation of free radicals, causing tissue damage and the outcome will be metabolic disorder. In such conditions, cleansing of channels (Srotoshodhana) is essential which is done by Panchakarma therapy.
- Bio-purification is potential in emergency conditions because only purificatory drugs possess the property of immediate action. Bio-purification is also administered in chronic poisoning. In the current era also, a human being is more exposed to acute & chronic poisoning, pesticide, chemical preservatives, etc. So now also there is a great need for bio-purification at least twice a year to purify the body from these harmful substances. It has now been scientifically shown that a natural purification treatment can successfully eliminate environmentally toxic substances and pesticides from the body, without damaging side effects.
- In chronic diseases, these will be a severe vitiation of channels (Srotodushti), weakness of digestive fire (Agnimandya), improper nourishment of tissues, and decreased immunity (Ojokshaya), which warrants the purification of body, so that the nutrients, medicaments, and energy may flow freely in the system as earlier. For this bio-purification through Panchakarma is indicated.
- Chronic disease cannot be managed without the combined and judicious use of Panchakarma therapy and rejuvenation therapy (Rasayana).
- Bio-purification makes the biological system to return to normalcy & to rejuvenate rapidly & also facilitates the desired pharmacokinetic effect of therapeutic remedies administered thereafter. It eliminates toxins & stagnated excreta & metabolites

from the body, cleanses the macron& microchannels, maximizes the absorption & metabolism of nutrients & drugs, and helps in minimizing their dose & toxicity.

Panchakarma practiced as Dinacharya (daily regimen) and Ritucharya (seasonal regimen) leads to health.

Dinacharaya & Ritucharaya
- Balancing bio fire (Agni)
- Balancing Doshas
- Balancing tissues (Dhatus)
- Elimination of waste (Malas)
- Cleansing of channels (Srotas)
- Clarity of mind (Manas)

Contraindications for Panchakarma
1. Not obeying physician's advises, cruel, Jealous, psychically unstable
2. Very weak strength, severe waste of muscles, complete depletive therapy, just fasted
3. Symptoms of death, severe trauma
4. Weak digestive fire, exhausted, old aged, child, pregnant
5. Very obese and very thin

Preparation to Panchakarma

POORVA KARMA (PRELIMINARY PROCEDURES)

Before the actual procedure of purification, there are some essential procedures called as preliminary procedures (Poorvakarma); they prepare the body and make the bio-humors (Dosha) fit for smooth and easy elimination.

After the kindling of digestive fire (Deepana), digestion of indigested/intermediate matter (Pachana), oleation (Snehana) and sudation (Swedana), the bio-humors should be expelled from the nearest route at the proper time according to the strength of the disease and the patient. From this, it is clear that there are four pre-purification procedures viz. Deepana, Pachana, Snehana, and Swedana.

Need of Poorvakarma

The whole bio-purification procedure depends upon the proper mobilization of bio-humors from the periphery (Shakha) to GIT (Koshta), which is achieved with the help of oleation and sudation.

Emesis and purgation are the purificatory procedures against the normal physiological processes of the body. Anything against any physiological activity of the body is bound to aggravate the Vata bio-humor. Hence the lubricating, softening, pacification of Vata bio-humor, etc. properties help protect the body from the negative onslaught of Vata bio-humor.

Importance

- As in a vessel smeared with oil, waterfalls down without sticking to the vessel, similarly, Kapha and other morbid humor are expelled, out easily in a body that has undergone oleation therapy.

- As a fire makes the water in moist wood to trickle out from every pore, similarly sudation therapy causes the adhered, stagnant toxic matter to melt and flow out in a person who has been previously oleated.
- Just as the dirt of cloth is separated and washed by soap and water, so by oleation and sudation therapies, the toxic matter in the body is separated and washed out by purgation.
- Purifictory therapy given without oleation and sudation would destroy the body like the dried wood.

Bio-Fire Enhancer (Deepana)

Deepana means enhancing, kindling or igniting of digestive fire. The drug that kindles the digestive fire, but does not digest the indigested matter (Ama) is called Deepana. Deepana increases appetite and quantity of food intake.

Single drugs used for enhancing the digestive fire.
- Piper longum (Pippali)
- Rfit of piper longum (Pippalimula)
- Piper Chaba (Chavya)
- Plumbago zeylanica (Chitraka)
- Zingiber officinale (Shunthi)
- Garcinia pedunculata (amlavetasa)
- Piper nigrum (Mareeca)
- Carum roxburghianum (Ajamoda)
- Ferula narthex (Hingu)
- Cyperus rotundus (Musta)
- Cuminum cyminum (Jeeraka)

All these can be used alone or in combination in the form of powder, decoction, or tablet.

Use of Deepana Drugs

a) Before the internal oleation therapy
b) In case of inadequate emesis or purgation
c) After emesis & purgation, to enhance the diminished digestive fire

Concept of Hunger and Appetite

The sensation of desire to take food described as hunger and appetite. Hunger is a physical need for food. Appetite is a physic and emotional desire to eat and not always associated with the need for food. It is acquired and is probably dependent upon pleasurable past experiences associated with eating. Thus because of hunger, one may eat a wholesome meal which is fully adequate for his needs and because of appetite, add to it a dessert which is entirely unnecessary for as requirements are concerned.

Mode of action

a) The purported stomachic mechanism of action of these substances is to stimulate the appetite by increasing the gastric secretions of the stomach.
b) Stimulation of vagus nerve e.g. Pilocarpine controls the secretion of gastric juice.
c) Stimulation of Glasopharyngeal nerve which increases appetite juice.
d) Stimulation of fundus of the stomach.
e) Stimulation of pylorus of the stomach.

Digestive (Pachana)

Pachana means digestion. Pachana drugs do the digestion of undigested matter but not increase the
Pachana Karma is for the digestion of undigested matter and also detachment morbid bio-humors (Dosha) from the tissues and microchannels. If oils & fats given in humor associated with indigested matter (Ama) severe complications occur and it would destroy the body.

Drugs used for Pachana

- A decoction of zinger & coriander seeds 30ml thrice a day
- Powders of a zinger, cyperus rotundus, Tinospora Cordifolia (in equal ratio) in a dose of 3-6 Gms thrice a day with hot/warm water
- The ginger powder alone 2 Gms with hot/warm water

- Trikatu Churna 2-3 Gms of powder thrice a day with hot/warm water
- Chitrakadi Vati 2 tablet thrice a day with hot/warm water
- Sudharshana Churna 4 Gms to 6 Gms thrice a day with water
- Hingvashtaka Churna 3 Gms with half spoon thrice day ghee & warm water
- Sanjeevani Vati 250mg to 500mg thrice a day with warm water

Uses

a) Before internal oleation therapy (Snehana) for the digestion of intermediate matter (Ama)

b) In case of inadequate emesis or purgation

Mode of Action

- Stimulation of Vagus Nerve which secretes gastric juice in the cephalic phase.
- Stimulates duodenum which leads to the secretion of digestive enzymes & hormones
- Stimulates the liver to secrete bile
- Stimulates pancreas to secrete pancreatic juice

Summary of action of Pachana-Snehana-Swedana

Stage of Bio-humor	Poorvakarma needed
Deep-seated humors	Deepana, Pachana, Snehana, Swedana
Detached from the tissues but not moving towards GIT	Snehana and Swedana
Detached from the tissues and moving towards GIT	Snehana and Swedana
Bio-humors are in GIT & ready to expelled through the oral & anal route	Only massage & sudation

SNEHANA KARMA (OLEATION THERAPY)

Snehana internal and external, both are preparatory procedures of purification therapy. Also, Snehana acts as the main therapy when it is given to pacify specific diseases or for the nourishment of the body.

Properties of Snehana Dravya

Fluid, Subtle, unctuous, slimy, heavy, cold, sluggish and soft.

Importance of Snehana

1. To eliminate diseases, two types of treatment are advised in Ayurveda grossly i.e. bio-purification (Shodhana) and palliative (Shamana). The diseases eliminated by bio purification will not recur. Before adopting therapy it is necessary to do Snehana and Swedana The idea of Snehana and Swedana is to bring out vitiated bio-humors to a suitable state so that they be expelled out easily This stage is called as an excitation of bio-humor. After these preparatory procedures, consequently, the bio-humors in the periphery are brought to the GIT.

2. Snehana is the first line of treatment for Vata disease there is no other drug equivalent to Taila in the management of Vata Roga.

3. The person who takes Sneha regularly will get the following benefits- the kindling of Bio-fire, purification of the bowel, nourishment of body tissues, increases strength, increases complexion sturdiness of sense organs, delayed aging and lives for hundred years.

4. By proper intake of Sneha with Anna, the Agni becomes stable.

5. In pediatrics, the children are said to be always being oleated because they are fed mainly with fatty or viscous food like breast milk or cow s milk, ghee, etc. So they can be directly subjected to mild bio-purification therapy whenever necessary.

6. Our body has a special affinity towards oils & fats that's why the body is considered as the essence of oils & fats. A person rich in oils & fats in the body will not be susceptible to diseases like tuberculosis etc. arising from fat deprivation in comparison to the persons who are not so.

7. It also seems to act as a preservative. By seeing the evolution of Ayurvedic pharmaceutics it seems that the preservative properties of Sneha have made the ancient medical man to store herbs and organic matters in Sneha Dravyas like oil, ghee, etc. Before the advent of mineral & metallic formulations, ghee and oil preparations happened to be the most widely used formulation.

Thus is the best-suited Dravya for the body it is used before Shodhana to bring the bio-humors (Dosha) to Koshta. If Shodhana is done without the Snehana & Swedana, then severe exhaustion, weakness occurs leading to the aggravation of Vata, so Snehana & Swedana are advised before Shodhana.

Sneha Dravya: Source of oleation material

For the oleation purpose mainly four types of Sneha are used in Ayurvedic viz. ghee (Ghrita), oil (Taila), animal fat (Vasa) and bone marrow (Majja).

Vegetable oils

The oil extracted from the seeds of certain plants is used for Snehana sesame, mustard, castor, coconut, etc. Out of these, sesame oil is considered for imparting strength. Sesame oil due to its hot property pacifies Vata but does increase Kapha, improves strength and complexion, stabilizes the muscles and the Srotas.

Taila - sesame oil.

- Taste (Rasa) – sweet.
- Properties (Guna) – strong, heavy, oily.
- Potency (Virya) – hot.
- After digestion (Vipaka) – sweet.
- Specific action (Prabhava) – no.

General action: Mitigates Vata and Kapha, Increases Pitta.

Animal Source of Sneha

Milk, ghee, milk products, meat, fat and bone marrow, liver oil are animals of Sneha. Out of this ghee is the best and is most common in practice.

Ghee relieves vitiation of Pitta and Vata, nourishes Rasa and Shukra, clarity to voice and complexion and has laxative action. Further out of all the of Sneha, ghee, particularly cow's ghee is considered best. It is best because it has Yogavahi property ie. when it is medicated with other drugs having even opposite properties, it carries their properties, without losing its properties.

Ghee

- Taste (Rasa) – sweet.
- Properties (Guna) – heavy, oily, soft, subtle
- Potency (Virya) – cold.
- After digestion (Vipaka) – sweet.
- Specific action (Prabhava) – no.

General action: Mitigates Vata and Pitta, Increases Kapha.

Muscle fat (Vasa)

- Properties are similar to the meat of animals from which fat obtained.

Fat is scraped, boiled. Collect in other vessels the oil on the water surface while boiling. Heat collected oil to remove water and store it in a container without the reach of air.

Bone Marrow (Majja)
- Properties are similar to the meat of animals from which fat obtained.

Extract directly from the bones. Cook, it separates like Ghee. Filter and store in the container without air access.

Mahasneda.
 The combination of all the four Snehas: oil, ghee, fat and bone marrow.

Combination of Sneha:

- Yamaka Sneha: The combination of any two Sneha is known as Yamaka Sneha, for example, ghee + oil and so on.
- Trivrut Sneha: The combination of any three Sneha, for example, ghee + oil + bone marrow and so on.
- Maha Sneha: The combination of two or all the 4 Sneha.

These Sneha combinations are used both internally and externally in the combination of two or all three Dosha.

Medicated oil & fat (Siddha Sneha)
These are the oils prepared with medicinal herbs. In classics, there are thousands of oils and ghee which are used extensively in various diseases with better therapeutic efficacy.

Fortified oil (Avartita Sneha)
It is a special type of oil prepared by repeated boiling of Sneha for 10, 100 or 1000 times with the decoction & paste of herbs. These are used in special conditions when the simple oil/ghee does not produce desired therapeutic results.

Properties

These oils can penetrate the microchannels of the body and used mainly in neurological disorders (Vata Vyadhi)

Indications

- Dreadful neurological disorders
- Neuropathy, Demyelinating disorders
- Degenerative diseases of joint, Chronic musculoskeletal disorders

Diet during Snehana

During the Snehana therapy, the patient is prescribed to take light to digest, warm and liquid diet containing only little fat. Any food that obstructs the Srotasa (Abhishyandi) should be avoided.

INTERNAL AND EXTERNAL SNEHANA

Based on a mode of application, oleation may be classified into two types oleation (Abhyantara Snehana), External oleation (Bahya Snehana).

Internal oleation (Abhyantara Snehana)

Indication of Internal Snehana

It is mandatory to perform Snehana as a part of preparatory measures before Panchakarma. It is very beneficial for Vata and its disorders. It is also indicated in persons who take diet deficient in fat (Ruksha) and who excessively indulge in sex, wine, exercise, and constant thinking. It is useful for children, aged, weak, for persons who have less body weight and patients with weak semen. It is also indicated in eye diseases like weak eyesight, blindness, and ptosis.

A dose of Sneha for Internal Snehana

The dose of Sneha is not mentioned directly in quantity; rather it is mentioned in terms of the digestive power of the individual patient. The quantity of Sneha digested in 24 hours is known as the maximum (Pravara) dose. The quantity of the Sneha digested in 12 hours is termed as medium (Madhyama) dose and the quantity of Sneha digested in 6 hours is considered as low (Hina) dose. Besides, a test dose (Hrasiyasi) has also been mentioned, which is the quantity of ghee digested within three hours of its intake. It is particularly useful for those cases where digestive power and Agni (Koshtha) is unknown.

A dose of Sneha:

- **Low dose** - The dose of the Sneha, which digests within 6 hours.

- **Medium dose** - The dose of the Sneha, which digests within 12 hours.
- **High dose** - The dose of the Sneha, which digests within 24 hours.

Types of Sneha According to Preparation:

- Mrudu Paka,
- Madhyama Paka,
- Khara Paka

Indications of the Sneha according to the type of Preparation

1. **Massage**: Khara or Madhyama
2. **Intake**: Madhyama or Mrudu
3. **Nasya**: Mrudu or Madhyama
4. **Basti**: Madhyama or Khara

Dosage strategy of internal oleation

Feature	Accha Sneha	Vicharana Sheha
Dose	High	Low
Stomach	Empty	Along with food
Effect	Quick and high	Slow and less
Restrictions	Obligatory	No need to follow
Complications	More chances	Rare
Purpose	Excitation and pacification	Nourishment and excitation
Merits	Best	Least

Contra Indication of Internal Snehana

1. Excessive Kapha and Meda (fat), obese.
2. Very weak, exhausted and unconscious persons
3. Pregnant ladies
4. Persons having persistent poor digestion or indigestion
5. Suffering from Udara Roga (diseases of the abdomen including those of liver, spleen, and ascites)
6. Slow poisoning or intoxication
7. Undergoing Basti and Nasya procedures
8. Just after Virechana procedures
9. Ama disorders
10. Diarrhea
11. Throat disorders (Gala Roga)
12. Abortion
13. Alcoholism.

Duration of Snehapana

- The doses of Shodhana Sneha should be planned in such a way that the proper Snehana occurs in 3 to 7 days. Generally in Mridu Koshtha, Snehana of the patient occurs in three days, while it may take 7 days in Krura Koshtha persons. The Sneha should be administered once in a day until the symptoms of proper Snehana are achieved. But Sneha should not be given beyond seven days because thereafter it becomes Satmaya (habitual) to the person and it will no longer work for Shodhana purpose. It means, if it is given beyond 7 days then it starts acting as a diet article and its drug value ceases.

- The main therapeutic action of Shodhana Sneha is to excite the Dosha so that they are taken out by Shodhana.

Goals of Sneha:

1. Palliative Oleation (Shamana Snehana)
2. Preparatory Oleation (Shodhanartha Snehana)
3. Instant oleation (Sadya Snehana)
4. Nutritive Oleation (Brimhana Snehana)
5. Purificatory Oleation (Shodhana Snehana)

Shamana (Palliative) Snehana

The medicated Sneha ghee or oil is administered orally for relieving various disorders. For example, Pancha Tikta Ghrita is administered orally as a part of palliative treatment of skin diseases, Pancha Gavya Ghrita is used in epilepsy, and Kalyanaka Ghrita is prescribed in psychiatric diseases and Bala Taila for Vata disorders. This Shamana Sneha is administered on an empty stomach at mealtime on getting the appetite in a medium dose.

Shamana Sneha is the administration of Sneha in different disorders to normalize the aggravated bio-humors without expelling them and disturbing the normal bio-humors.

It is a procedure of administration of a moderate dose of Accha Sneha during mealtime when one feels hungry in an empty stomach.

All the Sneha mentioned under the heading of Medicated oils & fats are used for palliative purposes.

Shodhanartha (Preparatory) Snehana

The Sneha administered internally for the preparation of the patient for Shodhana is termed as Shodhana Snehana. For this purpose, generally plain (Achchha) Sneha but occasionally disease wise medicated Sneha is administered orally in high dose, once in the morning, after the digestion of a meal taken on the previous night.

Sadya Snehana (Instant oleation)

Sometimes it becomes necessary to oleate a patient urgently. The administration of Sneha mixed with salt enhances the process of Snehana and is useful for instant (Sadya) Snehana. Children, elderly persons and people who are unable to follow the prescribed rules of oleation, may receive some benefits of Snehana by eating any of the following according to their constitution and disease.

Sadyosnehana is a procedure of administration of Sneha to achieve oleation instantaneously or within a shorter duration (within 3 days). It is based on the principles of Vicharana Snehana.

It is a type of abhyantara Sneha where Sneha Dravya is used in combination with dietary preparations. Medicated and non-medicated Sneha Dravyas can be used.

Indications of Instantaneous Oleation:

- Child, Elder person
- Decreased strength
- Weak digestive fire
- Exhausted by coitus
- Less humor
- Not able to follow the restrictions of oleation therapy
- Whenever immediate bio-purification (Shodhana) is intended
- Usually done as a preparatory procedure in bronchial asthma

Contra-indications of Instantaneous Oleation:

In diseases of the skin, diabetes mellitus and edema SadyoSnehana should not be given with aquatic meat, milk, Jaggery, curd, and sesamum.

Nutritive Oleation

The administration of Sneha along with meat soup, beer, milk, etc. is known as Brimhana Snehana. The dose of Sneha should be less.

Nutritive oleation is indicated in a child, elder, those suffering from thirst who dislikes oils & fat, alcoholic, takes oils & fats regularly, weak digestive fire, thin, fearful, soft bowel fewer humors and hot season.

The relation between Nutritive oleation time and food:

Before food

- Gives strength to lower limbs and low back.
- Downward movement of Vata,
- Cures diseases of lower limbs.

With food

- Enhances digestive fire
- Gives strength and stability
- Pacifies the abdominal pain.

After food:

- Enhances stability of sense organs
- Cures disorders of Head and Neck.

Purificatory Oleation (Shodhana Snehana)

The medium dose of oil/fat which is given in an empty stomach, when the person not having a hunger and the meal of the previous night is completely digested is said as purificatory oleation. Oleation used as a preparatory procedure of bio-purification is called purificatory oleation.

All the Sneha mentioned under the heading of Medicated oils & fats are used for palliative purposes.

Symptoms of Proper Oleation (Samyaka Snehana)

- Regulation of flatulence
- Improvement of digestion
- Unctuous and loose stool
- Unctuousness and softness of the body

Symptoms of Under Oleation (Asamyaka Snehana)

- Dry and hard stool
- Insufficient regulation of Vata
- Poor digestion and persistence of roughness
- Dryness of the body

Symptoms of Excessive Oleation (Ati Snehana)

- Heaviness
- Dullness
- Anorexia
- Nausea
- Unformed stools
- Pallor and
- Drowsiness

Classic oils for internal use

Name of the Sneha	Indication
Ardraka Ghrita	Abdominal pain
Ashtanga Ghrita	Mental retardation
Baladi Ghrita	Neurological disorders
Basti-Amayantaka	Renal and urinal diseases
Brahmi Ghrita	Psycho-emotional disorders
Darvibaladi Ghrita	Bleeding piles

Dhanvantara Ghrita	Diabetes
Dhanvantaram Taila 101	Neuro-muscular problems and pain
Guggulutiktaka Ghrita	Joint pain and back pain
Ikshuduradi Ghrita	Bleeding diseases
Indukanta Ghrita	Abdominal pain, ulcer⍰
Jivantyadi Ghrita	Refractive error
Kalyanaka Ghrita	Psycho-emotional disorders
Kooshmanda Ghrita	Emaciation
Ksheerabala 101	Neuro-muscular problems and pain
Mahakalyanaka Ghrita	Psycho-emotional disorders
Mahakooshmanda	Weak immunity
Mahapaishachika Ghrita	Weakness⍰
Mahatiktaka	Skin diseases
Marmakshata Ghrita	The trauma of vital points⍰
Pancagavya Ghrita	Neurological and Psycho-emotional disorders
Sarva Amayantaka Ghrita	Neurological disorders
Shatavaryadi Ghrita	Renal and urinal diseases
Tiktaka Ghrita	Skin diseases
Triphaladi Ghrita	Refractive errors

Algorithm of internal oleation

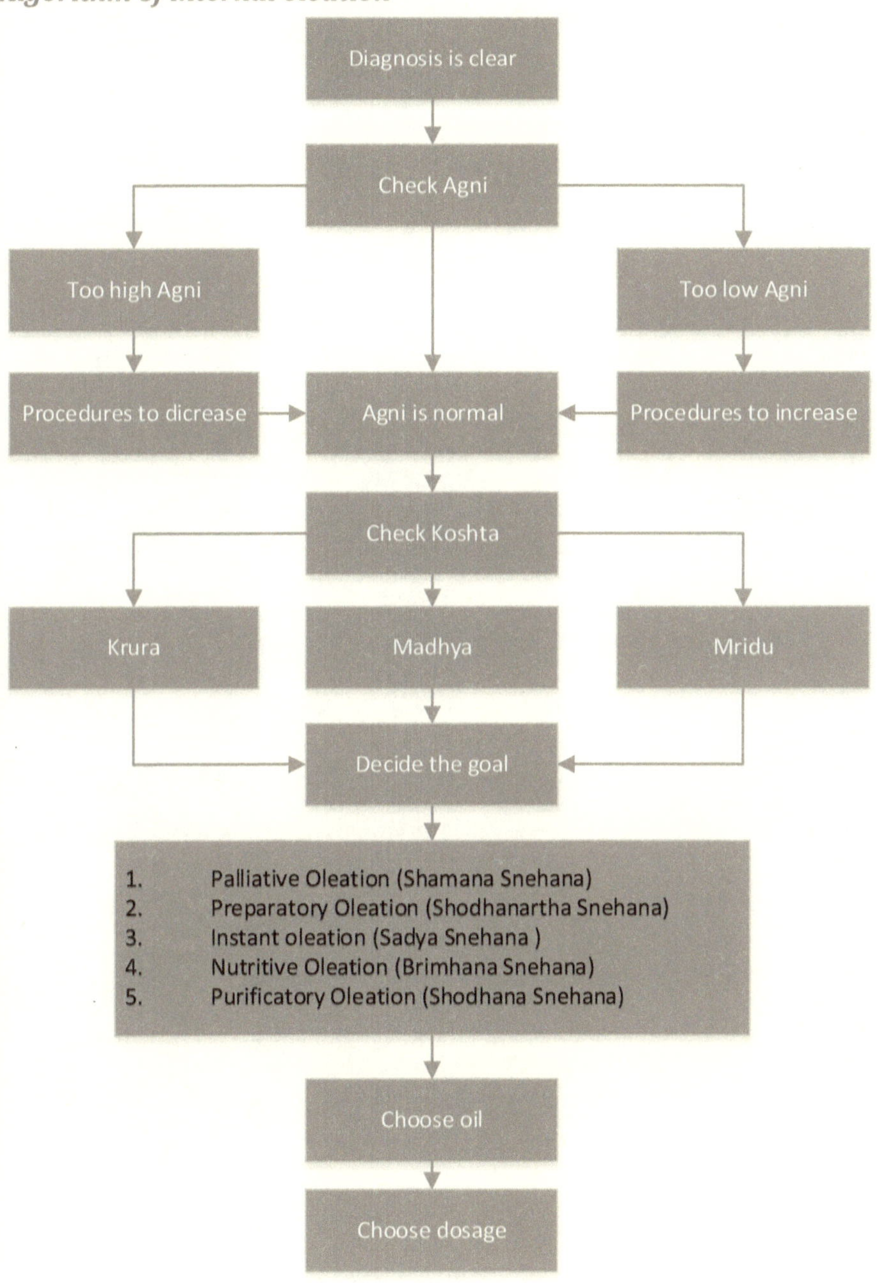

External Oleation: Bahya Snehana

Bahya Snehana means the external application of Sneha (plain or medicated). The common way of application is in the form of Abhyanga (massage). For performing this procedure the condition of the person and status of Dosha must be taken into consideration.

Indications of external Snehana

1. Exertion due to excessive physical work.
2. Habitual consumption of large amounts of liquor.
3. Excessive sexual activities.
4. Stress and Strain.
5. Suffering from Insomnia.
6. Patients of diseases such as Paralysis, Arthritis, Sciatica, Facial palsy, Backache, etc.
7. For people who are going to receive Swedana

Therapeutic considerations

1. Prakriti (constitution)
2. Dosha aggravation
3. Dhatu (tissues)
4. Roga (disease)
5. Rogi (patient)
6. Time
7. Region

Pharmacological considerations

1. Nature of drug
2. Dosage
3. Application frequency
4. Way of implementation
5. Anatomic variations & topical therapy
6. Epidermal barrier & rate of absorption
7. The temperature of oil & Hydration
8. Cost

Methods of External Oleation

Each of them has indications and contraindications.

- Abhyanga (Oil body massage)
- Shiro Abhyanga (Head massage)
- Vital points massage (Marma massage)
- Peep pressure massage (Mardana-Unmardana)
- Massage by foot (Padaghata)
- Gentle massage (Samvahana)
- Pouring of oil (Sneha parisheka)
- Tube oleation (Avagaha Sneha)
- Oral oil filling (Gandusha)
- Oil gargling (Kavala)
- Ears filling (Karnapurana)
- Eyes filling (Akshi tarpana)
- Scalp application (Tala & Talapotichil)
- Head oleation (Moordha taila & Shira tarpana)
- Poring on the forehead (Shirodhara, Takradhara & Ksheeradhara)
- Oiled cloth application on the head (Shiropichu)
- Oil bath for the head (Shirobasti)
- Oil bath on the back (Kati Basti)
- Oil bath over the cardiac region (Hrid Basti)
- Oil bath over the knees (Janu Basti)
- Palm massage (Mardana)
- Plucking massage (Unmardana)
- Powder massage (Udwartana)

Algorithm of external oleation

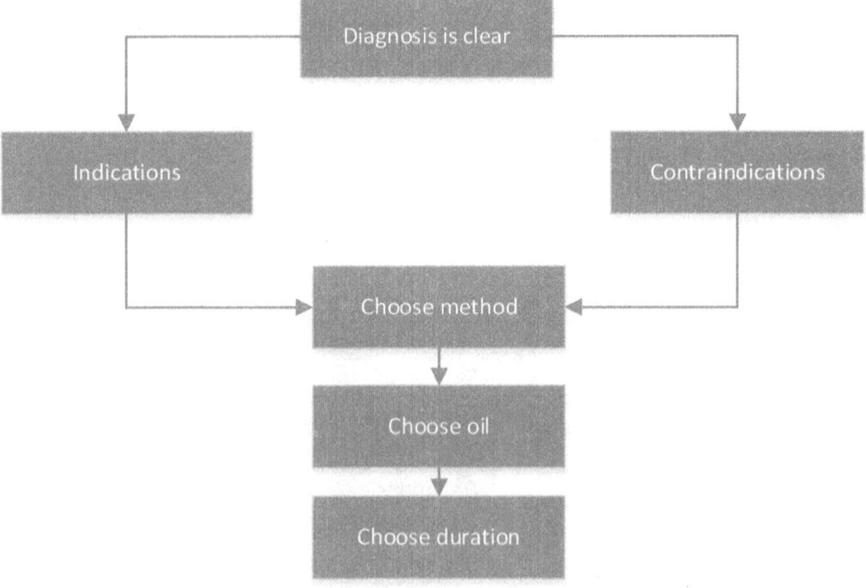

Commonly used oils for external oleation

Oil	Indication
Amrutottara Thaila	Wasting, chronic fever
Asanabilvadi Thaila	Head diseases
Bala Thaila	Neurological disorders
Balaguducyadi Thaila	Vascular diseases
Balashvagandi Thaila	Vata diseases
Bhringaraj Thaila	Hair problem
Dhanvantara Thaila	Vata diseases, back pain
Durdurapatradi Thaila	Hair problem
Durvadi Thaila	Skin diseases
Gandhaka Thaila	Skin diseases
Himasagara Thaila	Headache, insomnia
Jatyadi Thaila	Wounds
Karpasasthyadi Thaila	Paralysis
Kshirabala Thaila	Vata diseases, back pain
Maha Marichyadi Thaila	Skin diseases
Maha Mashadi Thaila	Paralysis, neuro-muscular problems
Mahanarayana Thaila	Paralysis, neuro-muscular problems
Mahavishagarbha Thaila	Painful Vata diseases
Murivenna Thaila	Skeleto-ligament problems
Neelibhringyadi Thaila	Hair problem
Panchaguna Thaila	Painful Vata diseases
Pinda Thaila	Vascular diseases
Sahacharadi Thaila	Vata diseases, back pain
Lakshadi Thaila	Vata diseases, Skeleto-ligament problems
Bilva Thaila	Ear pain
Apamarga Kshara Thaila	Ear pain
Guduchi Thaila	Psoriasis

SWEDANA KARMA (SUDATION THERAPY)

Sudation therapy is the next important preparatory procedure of Panchakarma therapy. Also, it is an important major therapy for the treatment of many diseases. Sudation therapy is a specific treatment for some Vata & Kapha predominant diseases.

Sudation therapy is the best treatment for vitiated Vata and Kapha dominant diseases. It is done to liquefy the oleated bio-humors brought about by oleation therapy.

The properties attributed to Swedana are Ushna (Hot), Tikshna (Sharp), Sara (Mobile), Drava (Liquid), Snigdha (Unctuous), Ruksha (Dry) and Sukshma (Subtle).

Definition

Swedana is defined as the procedure, in which the sweat or perspiration is produced in the body by using various methods. Swedana is the procedure, which relieves stiffness, heaviness, and coldness of the body and produces sweating.

Importance

Proper sudation administered after oleation therapy pacifies the Vata. By this, the feces, urine, and semen do not stagnate in the body. By application of oil followed by sudation therapy, the dry stick becomes soft and elastic. Then how will be its effect in an alive human being? means Swedana therapy will be having definitive therapeutic action.

Generally, fomentation is done once daily preferably in the morning hours on empty stomach for 21 days. If necessary the courses may be repeated with the interval of two to three weeks depending upon the tolerance of the person to the Swedana therapy.

Indications of Swedana

Swedana is indicated in Vata and Kapha disorders and before the Shodhana therapy. Its other main indications are the common cold, cough, pharyngitis, dyspnea, pain in ear, neck, and head; distension of abdomen, constipation; Ama disorders, colicky pain in the abdomen, feeling of heaviness, body ache; stiffness of flanks, back, waist and abdomen; pain and stiffness in foot, knee, thigh, and calf; osteoarthritis, sciatica, contracture, hardness, stretching, stiffness, numbness, cramps, tremors, paralysis, dysarthria, monoplegia, hemiplegia, dysuria, anuria, and inflammation.

Contraindication of Swedana

The sweating therapy is contraindicated in habitual alcohol drinker, pregnant lady, bleeding disorders, diarrhea, dehydrated persons, diabetes mellitus, anal fissure, prolapsed rectum, disorders due to excessive alcohol intoxication and poisoning, exhaustion, unconsciousness, excessive obesity, thirst, excessive hunger, anger, grief, jaundice, disorders leading to generalized enlargement of abdomen, tuberculosis, gout, weakness, fainting, and glaucoma. Affected with anxiety, Erysipelas, Fainting, Affected with sorrow, Fearful, Fracture, Alcoholic disease, menses, wound, Increased biological fire, Vata obstructed by Kapha & media -sudation without using fire

BENEFITS OF SUDATION THERAPY

1. Liquefaction of Dosha. Sudation therapy liquefies the vitiated bio-humors and directs them towards GIT.
2. Regulation of Vata- Proper regulation of Vata Dosha is important as it is the main factor responsible for controlling various activities of the body.

3. Relaxation of body parts- With the administration of proper Oleation and Sudation therapy, the body becomes soft and it attains elasticity.

4. The kindling of digestive fire.

5. Softening & cleansing of the skin. The skin contains numerous sweat glands, which when activated through sudation therapy excrete various toxic substances of the body in the form of sweat. As a result, the skin becomes soft and its texture improves.

6. Increases appetite- it improves appetite by digesting the indigested/intermediate matter.

7. Cleansing of channels- Sudation therapy induces cleansing of channels by dilating the openings of sweat glands and by regulating Vata bio-humor. As a result, stagnant waste, sweat, and various toxins are eliminated out of the body resulting in the cleansing of channels.

8. Alleviates excess sleep & stupor- Aggravated Kapha causes excessive sleep and drowsiness. Sudation pacifies Kapha and helps in relieving excessive sleep & drowsiness.

9. Mobility of J 0ints- Mobility of joint activity is regulated by the proper functioning of Vata & Kapha. For controlling, Vata & Kapha oleation followed by sudation therapy is best.

10. Purifies bio-humor Oleation therapy produces moistening of which are then liquefied by sudation therapy. These liquefied bio-humors brought into GIT and finally removed from the body.

Swedana done in the properly oleated patient excretes out the metabolic waste and harmful substances (Mala) situated in the subtle channels by melting and dissolving them. Snehana loosens the Dosha to some extent. The Swedana performed thereafter liquefies the Dosha situated in Dhatu at their place or elsewhere in the subtle channels and facilitates their bringing to Koshta by a respective measure of bio purification.

Other therapeutic actions of Swedana include improvement in appetite and digestion, softening of the skin, improvement in complexion as well as functions of the skin. Opening and cleansing of the microchannels relieves excessive sleep, laziness, drowsiness, stiffness of the joints, heaviness and cold, restores the normal function of the joints and excretes out the harmful toxins and metabolites along with sweat.

CLASSIFICATION OF SWEDANA

Based on the use of fire:

- Sudation with fire (Sagni Sweda)
- Sudation without fire (Anagni Sweda)

Based on Properties of the drug used:

- Unctuous sudation (Snigdha Sweda)
- Dry sudation (Ruksha Sweda)

Based on Modes of heat:

- Dry heat (Tapa Sweda)
- Steam bath (Ushma Sweda)
- Tub bath (Drava Sweda)
- Poultice (Upanaha Sweda)

Based on the site of Sweda:

- Local sudation (Ekanga Sweda)
- Generalized sudation (Sarvanga Sweda)

Based on potency

- Mild sudation (Mridu Sweda)
- Medium sudation (Madhya Sweda)
- Strong sudation (Maha Sweda)

Based on the type:

- External sudation (Bahya Sweda)
- Internal sudation (Abhyantara Sweda)

Based on the action:

- Palliative sudation (Samshamana Sweda)

- Purificatory sudation (Samshodhana Sweda)

Sudation without the fire used in cases:

- Exercise
- Indwelling in a warm chamber
- Wearing of heavy clothing
- Hunger
- Excess drinking
- Fear
- Application of poultice
- Anger
- Wrestling
- Exposure to sun rays

a) Palliative sudation (Samshamana Sweda): The Swedana used for digestion of bio-humors associated with intermediate matter and for the pacification of Dosha is called as Samshamana Sweda. It improves the power of Agni, skin becomes tender and delicate and it does the cleansing of microcirculatory channels.

b) Purificatory sudation (Samshodhana Sweda): This 1S used before bio purificatory therapies like Vamana, Virechana, etc. The main object of this type of sudation is to bring unctuous bio-humors from the periphery to GIT, from there the vitiated bio-humors are expelled out by appropriate Shodhana Karma.

Some consideration for choosing the method of sudation⬚
Season:

- Winter season- strong sudation
- Hot/summer season- Mild sudation

Rogi (patient):

- Good strength—strong sudation
- Medium strength - moderate sudation
- Less strength - mild sudation

Region:

- Tropical region - mild sudation
- Forest region- heavy or strong sudation
- Temperate region - moderate sudation

A body part:

- The heart region, testis, and eyes should be given mild sudation or as far as possible these regions should be avoided.
- Groins and lower abdomen should be given moderate sudation. For other parts

Swedana should be done up to the desired extent, means till the observation of adequate symptoms of sudation.

Administration of sudation:

- After considering the strength of the patient etc. as discussed above, suitable Sudation should be done to the patient who has undergone massage in a place devoid of air.
- The heat or steam should be checked by the therapist before applying or directing the patient to prevent the over sudation or burn wound.
- The sudation should be done in the vertical form at limbs and circular form at joint places.
- The sudation should be continued until the appearance of adequate symptoms of sudation, which has been described below.

Preparation of the patient: The sudation therapy is administered to a person whose last meal has been well digested and in a place free from wind. Always the patient's body should be massaged with oil before the sudation therapy (except in cases of acute fever, a condition associated with indigested matter, obesity, etc.).

Symptoms of adequate Swedana

Fomentation should be done continuously until the symptoms of proper Swedana appear:

1. Appearing of sweat
2. Relief in cold
3. Relief in heaviness
4. Relief in pain
5. Relief in stiffness
6. The softness of the skin.

Symptoms of inadequate Fomentation

1. Less sweating
2. NO relief from pain
3. No relief from cold
4. Stiffness in the body
5. Heaviness in the body
6. The roughness of the body

If there are symptoms of insufficient fomentation continue the process until the patient gets proper symptoms.

Symptoms of excessive Swedana

1. Aggravation of blood
2. Aggravation of Pitta Dosha
3. The appearance of blisters eruptions⬛
4. Burning sensation in the body
5. Fainting
6. Feeble voice
7. Fever

8. Heaviness or pain in the body
9. Pain in joints
10. Tiredness
11. Vertigo
12. Vomiting
13. Weakness

Management of complications of Swedana

If there are any symptoms of excessive fomentation, manage the complications by giving Madhura Rasa (Sweet taste), Snigdha (Unctuous), Drava (Liquid) and Shita (Cool) Guna (attribute) drugs and diet to the patient and also follow the regimen of Grishma Ritu (Summer season). Following measures should also be adopted:

1. Shita Mantha (A type of groat mingled with cold water and ghee) added with sugar
2. Shrita Shita Ialapana (Boiled and cooled water)
3. Madya (Alcohol) in addicted persons
4. Chandana Pralepa (Application of sandalwood paste)
5. Fanning with Chandanodaka (Sandal water)
6. Dwelling in a cool room in the day time and moonlight during the night.
7. Avoid Lavana (Salt), Amla (Sour), Katu Rasa (Pungent taste) and Ushna Guna

Commonly Used Herbs for Sudation Therapy

Leaves of plants:

- Moringa olefera (Shzgru)
- Ricinus communis (Eranda)
- Boerhavia diffusa (Punarnava)
- Calotropis procera (Arka)
- Dolicos biflorus (Kulattha)

- Vitex Negundo (Nirgundi)
- Eucalyptus (Tailaparni)

The root of plants:

- Premna mucronata (Agnimanth)
- Aegle marmelos (Bilva)
- Oroxylum Indicum (Shyonaka)
- Stereospermum suaveolens (Patala)
- Gmelina Arborea (Kashmiri)
- Desmodium gangeticum (Shaliparni)
- Uraria picta (Prushniparni)
- Tribulus Terrestris (Gokshur)
- Solanum Indicum (Bruhati)
- Solanum xanthocarpum (Kantakari)
- Sida cordifolia (Bala)

Panchakarma application

Will be in next publication